Contents

Key messages

- For thirty years, policy makers in the English NHS have attempted to devise financial incentive schemes to improve the performance of health services.

- Despite the disappointments, successive governments have remained convinced that their latest round of payment reform would finally create a self-improving health system.

- Over the last few years, the national NHS bodies have proposed new payment schemes to incentivise a single service provider or partnership of service providers to deliver high quality integrated care for local populations.

- There appears to be broad agreement among technical advisors on this way forward, including creating whole population budgets, new incentive schemes to reward providers for good performance and new arrangements to transfer risk and reward to providers.

- This paper questions whether these latest incentive schemes will be any more successful than their predecessors. There are significant unresolved difficulties in applying the type of incentive scheme developed for accountable care in insurance-based health systems to tax-funded health systems with state-owned providers and limited choice of provider.

- While English policy makers have gravitated to the payment schemes for integrated care in insurance-based health systems, other countries with tax-funded healthcare have been heading in a different direction.

- A number of these countries are now foregoing complex financial incentive schemes in favour of partnership arrangements between funders and planners and groups of service providers, with the focus on effective joint working to make best use of healthcare resources.

- Commissioners and providers in many local health systems in England have also now started the transition from arm's length contracting to collaborative relationships.

- While these arrangements are at an early stage, there is emerging evidence of the benefits. Organisations across local systems are working together as a single team and resources that would in the past be consumed by contracting are now being used for improvement.

Introduction

At the start of the Second World War, the allied forces established military bases on the Melanesian islands northeast of Australia in the Pacific Ocean. A steady stream of cargo planes arrived, bringing clothing, weapons, tents and food. When the war was over, the native Melanesian tribes patiently re-enacted what they had seen, using bamboo and straw to construct replica runways, control towers, radar antennae and Nissen huts. For decades they lit signal fires along their runways at night, hoping, despite the repeated disappointments, that one day an aeroplane would arrive.

Over the last thirty years the English NHS has repeated a peculiar managerial ritual of its own: the development of payments, incentives and contracts to reward health services for performance. Despite the disappointments, successive governments remained convinced that their latest round of payment reforms would finally create a self-improving health system. The national NHS bodies now set prices for 3,000 services, from £63 for the simplest accident and emergency (A&E) attendances to £40,550 for the most complex intercranial operations. There are uplifts for complexity, carve-outs for high-cost inputs, caps for higher volumes and penalties for failed procedures. There are dozens of financial incentives to motivate performance, from cleaning in hospitals to adopting new technologies.

Each iteration of the ritual has ended in failure. Since the national tariff was introduced in the early 2000s, the NHS has struggled to set appropriate prices, rewarding or punishing organisations unfairly (PricewaterhouseCoopers 2012). Devised to increase activity, the tariff now undermines important objectives such as reducing the need for hospital services, reallocating resources to priority areas such as primary care and mental health and integrating care. Our current combination of piecework payments for hospitals and capitation or block contracts for primary and community care incentivises the wrong things in the wrong places: treatment rather than prevention, care in hospital rather than closer to home. Meanwhile, there is little evidence that incentive schemes such as the Commissioning for Quality and Innovation (CQUIN) framework have delivered substantial improvements in quality or efficiency (Thomas 2018; Forbes *et al* 2017).

Nevertheless, the enthusiasm for complex new payment schemes remains unabated. As the problems associated with payment for individual procedures became clear, the NHS started experimenting with payments and incentives for larger bundles of services: first, whole pathways of care such as musculoskeletal or maternity services; then groups of services for subgroups of the population such as the frail elderly or people with mental health challenges; and now whole population budgets to deliver a broad range of health and care services in a local area (*see* Figure 1). In its consultation documents on the draft integrated care contract of 2018, NHS England explains how commissioners can bring together a 'whole population annual payment' and contract with a single integrated care provider to deliver services for a local

Figure 1 Main payment mechanisms for health services

Cost pass-through	Fee-for-service	Bundles	Capitation	Block
This system involves paying costs providers incur for services.	This system involves paying a fixed price for each unit of activity.	This system involves paying a fixed price to manage the care of a particular pathway of care.	This system involves payment of a fixed sum per capita to provide a range of services to a particular population.	Lump sum payments are made to individual providers to provide a group of services to a particular population in this system.
This could include reimbursing providers' costs for high-cost devices or drugs, or reimbursing providers' estates costs, for example.	This could include fixed tariffs for A&E attendances, elective operations and particular tests, for example.	Tariffs for the maternity pathway or hip replacement and rehabilitation might be bundled, for example.	It often includes incentive payments for performance.	There is typically no systematic change to reflect population size of payments linked to outcomes.
	Fee-for-service systems are sometimes combined with incentive payments for specific aspects of performance such as under the Commissioning for Quality and Innovation (CQUIN) framework.	Typically, this system includes payments or penalties to reflect performance, for example penalties for complications or readmission to hospital after surgery.		For example, block grants would be given in mental health and community services.

population. As part of this, it proposes a new 'incentives framework' to motivate performance and new 'gain/loss sharing' arrangements to 'build and align financial incentives across local areas' (NHS England 2018c). NHS England is now considering the use of payments and incentives in the development of primary care networks and other priorities set out in the NHS long-term plan (NHS England 2019).

There appears to be broad agreement among technical advisers on this way forward. Advisers in management consultancies, as well as some research organisations, have recommended a move to capitation for local systems combined with other payment mechanisms, gain/loss sharing arrangements and incentive payments for meeting system-wide targets (Lewis and Agathangelou 2018; PricewaterhouseCoopers and Healthcare Financial Management Association 2018). Some argue that the payment systems for integrated care must inevitably be 'far more complex' than simply moving to capitation, with 'the potential for multiple payer relationships and forms of payment' (Lewis and Agathangelou 2018). Non-experts have struggled to penetrate discussions dominated by the technical incantations of accountable care in the United States: 'value-based payments', 'upside and downside risk', 'unbalanced and asymmetric risk sharing' (Wyatt 2018). Most of us aren't entirely sure what all the terms and formulae mean.

This paper questions whether these latest incentive schemes, borrowed in large part from the contractual models for accountable care in the United States, will be any more successful than their predecessors. It starts with a brief summary of the history of financial incentives in the NHS, highlighting the tendency to repeat the same unsuccessful experiments. It then provides a review of recent incentive schemes for large groups of local services. Most of our critique could apply directly to any of the incentive schemes tried in the NHS in the last few years, for example, the unsuccessful UnitingCare Partnership contract for older people's services in Cambridgeshire and Peterborough, the troubled contract for older people's services in East Staffordshire, or incentive schemes for particular national priorities. The final sections outline an emerging alternative approach.

Our objections to these latest schemes are partly technical. One recurring challenge is how to measure the performance of health services as a basis for handing out financial rewards and penalties. As experience has shown, it is extremely difficult to devise metrics that effectively capture local health systems' overall performance and can be measured accurately in the short to medium term. Another recurring challenge is how to apply financial incentives effectively in public health systems. If the state withholds payments from underperforming health care providers, this makes it harder for them to deliver adequate services: the absurdity of punishing patients who have already been let down by risking even worse care (Illman 2018). In practice, the state often bails struggling providers out, undoing the intended effects of the incentive scheme.

Our objections are also partly philosophical. If the aim of introducing financial incentives in the NHS was to inject the dynamism of markets, the result so far has been quite the opposite. For Hilary Cottam, financial incentives in public services are 'a modern version of command and control', rewarding staff 'like children, with pocket money' (Cottam 2018). While economists might calculate the considerable transaction costs, it is hard to put a figure on the wider consequences, for example, the local leaders locked in recriminations about targets and payments rather than developing more constructive, collaborative approaches to the stewardship of local systems (Ham and Alderwick 2015). Most pernicious of all is the capacity of this modern bureaucracy to blind public services to their true purpose: the collective anaesthesia that allows a foundation trust to put financial targets over compassion (Berwick 2013) or, in education, a grammar school to put its position in league tables above the wellbeing of its children (Millar 2018).

There is an alternative way forward. While English policy-makers have gravitated to the complex payment schemes for integrated care used in insurance-based health systems (Monitor 2014), other countries with tax-funded health care that is culturally and structurally much closer to the English NHS – Scotland, Sweden, New Zealand amongst others – have been heading in an entirely different direction. In New Zealand, the Canterbury District Health Board abandoned transactional approaches to managing its local health system in the late 2000s. Rather than engineering complex incentive schemes, it has focused on developing with providers a compelling vision for local services and the management systems needed to improve performance. Rather than attempting to transfer risk and reward to providers, it recognises the state's responsibility to run a stable public health system. Rather than devising algorithms to apportion gains or losses, it agrees with providers how to reallocate resources to meet the community's needs. This change of approach has allowed local leaders to build effective relationships and staff across services to work as a single team, while funds that would otherwise be consumed by contracting can now be used for quality improvement.

After more than thirty years of new public management in England, the belief that state funders should maintain arm's length relationships with public services and rely on financial levers to improve performance is now baked into the political and administrative consciousness. When particular rituals have been iterated for so long, it will always be difficult to abandon them and there will inevitably be anxiety about what will replace them. Nevertheless, commissioners and providers in many local health systems in England – Bolton, Leeds, South Tyneside among others – have now started the transition from arm's length contracting to collaborative relationships. These new approaches are evolving and vulnerable, but there is emerging evidence that they are delivering benefits. If such transformation is possible, it may be because these new ways of working are not entirely new. They reconnect with traditions of collaboration in public service that have been obscured temporarily but remain part of the NHS.

A clockwork universe

When the Stanford economist Alain Enthoven touched down in London in 1984, his brief from his sponsor, the Nuffield Provincial Hospitals Trust, was to review the management and organisation of health services in the United Kingdom as if he were 'a man from Mars' (Enthoven 1985). Confounded by the jargon of the NHS – 'At times I felt I could barely grasp the language' – he evidently felt well placed to offer an outsider's perspective. Beyond the confines of health services, city traders had caught sight of Motorola's DynaTAC 8000x, the size and weight of a bag of flour, making it the first 'handheld' mobile phone. Margaret Thatcher's battle with striking mineworkers was in full train, with ugly clashes on picket lines in the Midlands and Yorkshire. The Soviet Union, now indisputably on the rocks, was bankrupting itself with defence spending while relying on the United States for imported grain.

Enthoven's incisive 'reflections' on the NHS, published a year later, describe an 'entrenched bureaucracy' to match those crumbling soviet economies (Enthoven 1985). Ministers pursued short-term political expediency with little concern for running an efficient health system. The public servants responsible for overseeing health districts had little managerial expertise and even less leverage over services. Decisions were made, not in the public interest, but in the interests of unionised workers, the medical profession and providers. And, most importantly, there were 'no serious incentives to guide the NHS in the direction of better care and service at reduced cost'. Instead, efficient providers were punished with budget cuts, while inefficient services that ran up waiting lists were rewarded with bailouts. The result was a 'gridlock of forces that made change exceedingly difficult to bring about'. Closing a redundant hospital was about as easy as closing a redundant coal mine.

If these were the problems, Enthoven proposed a three-pronged solution: distancing politicians from the NHS; professionalising its management; and establishing a market in public health care. The Griffiths Inquiry had already recommended separating political oversight from the management of service delivery and the appointment of professional managers to oversee services. But Enthoven argued that these changes, while welcome, would be 'little more than cosmetic' unless they went hand in hand with market reforms, in particular giving health districts a fixed budget for their population, encouraging them to purchase from the most efficient providers, offering financial incentives to improve performance, using competitive tendering and allowing outsourcing to the private sector.

Four years later, Enthoven's recommendations were government policy. After the 1987 election, Margaret Thatcher convened a small ministerial group – Nigel Lawson, John Major, Ken Clarke and David Mellor – who met weekly to discuss health service reform. While scrupulously avoiding any direct mention of competition or markets, the 'Working for patients' White Paper of January 1989 recast district health authorities, not as managers in a public-sector hierarchy, but as purchasers of services on behalf of their populations. In language that would enter the lifeblood of the NHS, the health authorities could then 'concentrate on ensuring that the health needs of the population for which they are responsible are met', ensuring that the population had access to 'a comprehensive range of high quality, value for money services' and on 'setting targets and monitoring performance'. At the same time, hospitals would be encouraged to become new, self-governing 'hospital trusts' that would contract with different health authorities and enjoy greater freedom to manage their staff and services. Larger GP practices could apply to hold the budgets for a range of hospital services and obtain them from either the NHS or the private sector.

As we now know, these prescriptions would not be limited to or even primarily directed at health care. Instead, what emerged was a universal doctrine for public service reform, a 'public management for all seasons' that would be applied, by right-wing and left-wing governments alike, to a broad range of public services. For the social scientist Christopher Hood, it represented the marriage of two streams of 20th century thought: a particular brand of 'business-like managerialism' coupled with the new institutional economics' concern with replacing inefficient bureaucracies with responsive markets (Hood 1991). While the recipe was adapted, a common group of ingredients was almost always present: distancing government from service delivery; arm's length contracting with services; defining more explicit performance standards that focus on desired outcomes; encouraging more hands-on, professional management of services; promising managers greater freedom to decide how to deliver the desired outcomes and using financial incentives, choice and competition to motivate improvement (Hood 1995, 1991).

5

In the English NHS, we have spent the last three decades attempting to operationalise variants of the model – albeit with many fits, starts and changes of direction along the way. The third Thatcher government made an initial attempt to distance politicians from service delivery by creating a 'health services supervisory board', chaired by the Secretary of State, to provide political oversight of the health system, and an 'NHS management board', without political representation, responsible for policy implementation and controlling performance. As discussed above, it also made the first attempts to create arm's length purchasers, free providers from state control, and encourage purchasers and providers to trade in an internal market.

The Blair governments made renewed attempts to create independent purchasers by separating primary care trusts from community services, to empower providers by establishing foundation trusts, and to harness competition through payment reform and patient choice. In 2003, the Department of Health started to roll out the Payment by Results system, paying hospitals a flat fee for each service they provided, for example an A&E or outpatient visit or elective operation. In 2004, it introduced the Quality and Outcomes Framework (QOF) for primary care, paying GP practices up to 10 per cent of their income based on performance against around 80 indicators covering preventive care and management of long-term conditions. In 2009, it introduced the CQUIN framework, paying NHS trusts a small percentage of their income, based on whether or not they meet performance targets such as advising on smoking or treating sepsis. The Blair governments also built on earlier attempts to create a regulatory regime to support a market, for example establishing rules on anti-competitive conduct and controlling mergers.

When Andrew Lansley arrived at Richmond House in 2010, he launched yet another blueprint to prevent 'political micromanagement of the health service', this time by creating a new NHS commissioning board; he put forward yet another strategy to 'liberate' purchasers and providers, this time through creating GP-led clinical commissioning groups (CCGs) and giving foundation trusts new freedoms; and he presented yet another plan to establish the regulatory infrastructure for a market, this time by establishing an independent economic regulator. Like Enthoven's essay a quarter of a century earlier, the White Paper of 2010 lamented the 'absence of an effective payment system' to improve outcomes. Like Enthoven's essay, it argued for 'strong incentives to reward quality and efficiency'. Recognising that 'payment by results' had rewarded activity rather than quality, it promised a new payment system that will reward overall performance: 'Payment should reflect outcomes, not just activity, and provide an incentive for better quality.' 'Money will follow the patient through transparent, comprehensive and stable payment systems across the NHS to promote high-quality care, drive efficiency and support patient choice' (Department of Health 2010).

At the heart of these reforms, there is an enduring conviction that recalibrating financial incentives will have a predictable, mechanical effect on a complex system. As the systems thinker Jake Chapman puts it, they assume a simple, linear relationship between 'policy decisions, corresponding interventions and a set of consequences' (Chapman 2004). In this clockwork universe, smart people at the centre just need to pull the right levers and put in place appropriate supporting conditions to create a self-improving health system. The anthropologist James Scott has described how these top-down interventions, supposedly guided by scientific rationality, but in fact based on 'thin simplifications' of the systems in which they are being introduced, routinely have perverse consequences and end in failure (Scott, 1998).

Returning to the United Kingdom as a Nuffield Trust fellow in 1999, 15 years after his initial visit, Enthoven made a nuanced assessment of the reforms he had helped to set in motion. While maintaining that the internal market had delivered some benefits, he recognised that progress had been slow and tangible impact limited. This was in large part because the government had failed to lay the foundations for a market-based system: politicians did not distance themselves from the service; purchasers were not free to buy selectively; providers were not free to innovate; incentives were not properly reformed. Enthoven's description of the obstacles to progress might have been cut and paste from his earlier paper as if nothing had really changed. One difference is that the tone of self-assurance had evaporated: 'Creating a quasi-market that improves performance in a social service prone to market failure is a very complex matter, more complex than the government of the time thought, more complex than I had realised.' Nevertheless, in his final analysis, Enthoven clung to his earlier recommendations: 'The most practical way to move forward now is to build on the strengths of the internal market and try to correct the factors that held it back' (Enthoven 1999).

The emerging new payment model for integrated care

While the focus in the 1990s was on payments and incentives for individual health services, commissioners started in the 2010s to experiment with incentive schemes for larger groups of services. These included payment schemes for whole pathways of care, such as Bedfordshire CCG's contract with Circle Health to deliver musculoskeletal services, and for whole subgroups of the population such as Cambridgeshire and Peterborough CCG's contract with the UnitingCare Partnership to deliver services for adults and older people. In the summer of 2018, NHS England set out proposals for commissioners to bring together funding in a simplified capitated budget, a 'whole population annual payment', and contract with a single 'integrated care provider' to deliver a broad range of services for a defined local population (NHS England 2018a).

While these schemes bring together funding and services in ways that were not envisaged in the 1980s or 1990s, there are many similarities with Enthoven's and others' original prescriptions for commissioners contracting with independent providers in a market-based system. Commissioners are expected to determine appropriate outcome measures and tender to select the best provider to deliver services. At least in theory, commissioners are expected to give the provider freedom to decide how to deliver these objectives. 'It is for the integrated care provider to determine how best to allocate its budget in order to meet the requirements for short- and long-term improvements in population health set out by commissioners in the contract' (NHS England 2018d).

Like their predecessors, these latest contracting approaches pin their hopes on the payment system to incentivise good performance. According to NHS England, financial incentives are important to ensure 'investment in preventive care', 'treatment in the appropriate lowest cost setting', 'provider accountability for the holistic care needs of individuals' and 'collaboration across current provider boundaries'; 'Otherwise it can be very difficult for providers to work together to deliver outcomes for the system as a whole' (NHS England 2017). One feature of these schemes is for commissioners to hold back a proportion of the budget for payment only if certain performance standards are met. Another is to transfer a range of demand and operational risks from the commissioner to the provider (NHS England 2018b).

Focusing on outcomes

The proposal that commissioners should define high-level outcome measures and incentivise the provider system to deliver them is appealing in theory. In this latest iteration of the clockwork universe, commissioners just need to specify sufficiently broad outcome measures to motivate overall improvement. In its consultation on the integrated care provider contract, NHS England proposed high-level measures such as healthy life expectancy at birth, inequality in life expectancy, and social isolation (NHS England 2018b). With such measures, the hope is that providers will make astute decisions about how best to deploy resources and reconfigure services to improve overall population health.

In practice, we know that it is extremely difficult to define and measure high-level outcomes for complex groups of health and care services. As Sir Michael Marmot and others have shown, a range of socio-economic forces influence health and wellbeing (Marmot 2004). It is extremely difficult to extrapolate the relatively small contribution of health services to changes in life expectancy at birth or overall health. Others have shown that many of these high-level measures of health and wellbeing are subject to national or global trends (Raleigh 2018). Local systems should of course focus on improving these outcomes. But we are peering through frosted glass: the data may provide indications of whether we are on the right track, but it won't provide a precise assessment or a basis for handing out rewards or penalties. Don Berwick has described the frustration felt by staff when they receive rewards or penalties based on measures that do not reflect their performance or are outside their control (Berwick 1995).

Faced with these difficulties in using high-level measures of performance, it seems highly likely that commissioners will revert back to narrower metrics that are easier to measure and attribute to health services: adherence to process, delivery of outputs such as volume of activity, and outcomes for narrowly defined services.

(5)

The risks in using these types of measures have been well documented: focusing on procedural steps rather than the overall effectiveness of care; attending to the aspects of performance being incentivised and neglecting those that aren't; carrying out activities simply to secure payments; or maintaining outdated practices rather than developing new, more effective ways of meeting patients' needs. The stronger the incentives attached to faulty measures, the greater the risk of these unintended consequences.

Pay for performance

Even if commissioners could easily identify and measure appropriate outcome measures, there are other fundamental difficulties in using financial incentives in public health systems. The architects of these new schemes have clearly taken inspiration from the payment models for integrated care in insurance-based health systems, in particular the incentive schemes for accountable care organisations in the United States (Monitor 2014). However, there are significant differences between a tax-funded system with publicly owned hospitals and insurance-based systems with a wider range of independent service providers.

In the English NHS, unlike many insurance-based health systems, state funders contract with publicly owned, not-for-profit NHS providers for most services. There are no shareholders to receive dividends if the provider does well or suffer losses if it does badly. Nor do managers or clinicians receive substantial bonuses linked to the financial performance of the provider. Instead, a public-sector provider might build up a surplus to reinvest in services if it performs well or run up a deficit if it performs badly. If commissioners use financial incentives to reward providers who are performing well in these systems, they risk misallocating resources that could be better spent elsewhere in the health system. If they withhold payments from providers who are performing badly, they make it harder for these providers to deliver adequate services within budget, running the risk that patients receive even worse care.

In comparison with insurance systems, NHS commissioners also often contract with a relatively small number of local providers, who are often essential providers of services to their populations. Under emerging new contracting models, commissioners will transfer whole population budgets to organisations or partnerships bringing together a wider range of local services. Unlike insurance-based systems where there is a range of competing providers, the state will need to bail these providers out if they enter financial difficulty to protect access to care. There are few plausible solutions to this problem in health systems organised along the lines of the English NHS. Even full privatisation would not solve the problem, since the state would still rely on a limited number of essential providers to deliver key local services.

Allocation of risk and reward

One key feature of recent schemes is the careful allocation of different forms of risk between commissioners and the integrated care provider. Among proponents of the model, there is a consensus that the commissioner should bear the risk that the population grows and that health needs increase. Meanwhile, the integrated service provider should bear the risk that patients use services more than envisaged, that it fails to implement intended efficiencies, or that system-wide changes reduce the quality of care. Again, the inspiration for these proposals appears to come from insurance-based health systems, in particular the United States.

In insurance-based health systems, insurers take responsibility for population risk. They raise funds and transfer a larger budget to the integrated care provider to reflect population growth or higher health needs. Meanwhile, insurers have at least some hope of ensuring that providers bear operational risks, profiting if they manage those risks well and absorbing losses if they manage them poorly. In insurance-based systems, these agreements are of material importance, determining which party wins or loses and the conditions for profit-making.

In the NHS, commissioners are only in a position to take responsibility for population risk if the overall funding allocated to the NHS matches the demands placed on it. Meanwhile, as above, commissioners will find it hard to ensure that integrated care providers bear operational risks if they materialise. These are the monopoly providers of essential services that cannot easily be allowed to become bankrupt and exit the market. In public systems, the agreement on who bears which risk is in any case of less obvious importance. Commissioners and many providers are divisions of the public sector with, ultimately, a single balance sheet.

Gain/loss sharing agreements

In its consultation on the new integrated care provider contract, NHS England also advises commissioners to enter gain/loss sharing agreements with the integrated care provider and other service providers to determine how they will share the gains or losses from particular service improvement projects. It proposes a six-stage process for reaching these agreements, including projecting expected activity levels and costs and using logic models to determine how to distribute gains or losses. As the guidance explains, the distribution of potential gains or losses between participants should depend on the likelihood of generating gains or losses as well as different parties' ability to influence the risk and their ability and appetite to bear risk. 'This means that, as far as possible, shares should be more sophisticated than simple 50/50 shares or "in proportion to revenue" shares' (NHS England 2017).

Private firms sometimes need to enter complex agreements pinning down precisely how they will share profits or losses from joint ventures. It is less clear why commissioners and providers in the NHS would attempt to do so. It seems inconceivable that they will be able to reach detailed agreements on how to share savings from a vast array of improvement projects in local systems at the start of a 10- to 15-year contract. For the most part, these complex agreements only serve to apportion surpluses and overspends between different parts of the public sector. Moreover, it is far from clear that surpluses or overspends should be shared between public services according to their ability to influence a particular risk and their contribution to the outcome as proposed. Surely commissioners and providers should use profits as effectively as possible to improve overall patient care and absorb losses in ways that minimise damage to patient care and protect the sustainability of services?

Transaction and distraction costs

As we pick through these proposals, what becomes apparent is the significant costs and complexities of transactional approaches to managing local health systems. Commissioners must develop baseline assessments of population needs and the volumes, costs and quality of services. They must try to identify with providers the vast range of areas for improvement at the start of the contract and make projections of how activity levels, quality and costs might change. They must measure large numbers of metrics as a basis for handing out rewards or penalties, with limited confidence that they will provide an accurate measure of performance. The data requirements are enormous, going well beyond what is needed for improvement. While there is limited information on the costs of NHS contracting, we know that establishing these types of contracts can cost many millions of pounds (National Audit Office 2016).

There is a direct relationship between the use of financial incentives, attempts to neatly apportion risk and reward and the costs of transacting with providers (Bajari and Tadelis 2001). When commissioners seek to harness financial incentives, it becomes important to pin down the circumstances in which payments should be made or withheld. When commissioners seek to transfer risk and reward, they must develop contracts that prevent providers escaping those risks if they transpire, for example cutting their losses by terminating the contract early. They need to specify how the parties will deal with changing circumstances, for fear that they will use changes as an excuse for reneging on commitments or renegotiating the deal. In short, they find themselves attempting to write complete contracts that cover every eventuality, a costly and ultimately futile endeavour for complex services over 10- to 15-year periods.

One consequence of the use of financial incentives is that commissioners find themselves pitted against providers in profoundly adversarial relationships. The leaders of the system spend large amounts of time in confrontational discussions about whether standards were met and whether it is reasonable to make or withhold incentive payments. Each party plays the system to protect its own financial position. Each party blames external factors if performance slips: the population's needs were more significant than predicted; the projections were unrealistic; the requirements changed; other organisations didn't do what was expected of them. When we attempt to pin down responsibilities in detailed contracts, collaboration becomes increasingly difficult. Anything that is omitted from the contract is discretionary. Anything that falls outside an organisation's direct responsibility is unlikely to be treated as a priority.

A shifting landscape

It is impossible to ignore the disparity between these proposals and other national policies. On the one hand, NHS England and NHS Improvement are working in closer partnership; their regional teams are focusing less on the positions of individual organisations and more on the sustainability of local systems;

government has reasserted control of foundation trusts; the provider sustainability fund is being used to protect the financial positions of providers; the failure regime for foundation trusts was abandoned after the administration process for Mid Staffordshire NHS Foundation Trust; and NHS Improvement appears to have largely abandoned economic regulation. On the other hand, current guidance insists that commissioners should contract on an arm's length basis with providers to deliver integrated care, deploying the incentives of markets and seeking to transfer risk and reward to the provider sector, as if Andrew Lansley's model of independent purchasers and providers remained perfectly intact.

One explanation is that the national NHS bodies are hamstrung by legislation: they cannot simply redefine the roles of commissioners or abandon procurement rules established in the Health and Social Care Act 2012. However, there also appears to be some lack of recognition of how much the world has changed and the extent of the implications for the traditional commissioning model. The purchasing model for improving health services, with its focus on financial incentives and risk transfer, was only ever likely to deliver benefits in the context of patient choice and an increasingly diverse and independent provider sector. While these conditions have never existed in the NHS, there have in the past been plans to develop them. In a health system where services are, for good reason, being brought together in integrated systems and where policies to encourage choice of provider and provider independence are largely in abeyance, the tools of arm's length purchasing look increasingly redundant.

Beyond the world of public health care, the arm's length contracting model for managing public services and regulating monopolies is also under scrutiny. In education, many are now arguing that encouraging schools to pursue narrow measures of performance may be doing more harm than good (Millar 2018). In transport, there is increasing criticism of the arm's length contracting model for overseeing rail franchises (House of Commons Transport Committee 2017). In water, there is a fierce debate on the merits of economic regulation of private providers versus public or community ownership (Ford and Plimmer 2018).

Different tools

Canterbury District Health Board, New Zealand

In November 2009, the Canterbury District Health Board took possession of a large, disused warehouse on the outskirts of Christchurch, New Zealand, and staff began to wheel hospital beds, surgical equipment, sheets of cardboard and household furniture into the building. Over the next six weeks, more than 2,000 doctors, nurses, managers and members of the public arrived at the warehouse. They began by discussing the strengths and weaknesses of the local health system before walking through mock-ups of hospital wards, health centres and people's homes, their brief to design the system they would want to rely on in future. Outside the warehouse with its cardboard cut-outs, the bricks and mortar health system was collapsing. In 2006, some 5,000 people had been dropped from waiting lists for operations and denied care. They might have wondered if this elaborate role play was the best use of everybody's time.

The Canterbury District Health Board's approach to transforming its local health and care system has now been carefully documented (Charles 2017; Timmins and Ham 2013). The 'showcase' event in the warehouse and other similar exercises in the late 2000s led to a set of high-level statements on how organisations should work together and ambitions for improving services. Over the next decade, clinicians and managers across the region pursued dozens of projects to strip out waste and improve how services worked together (Gullery and Hamilton 2015).

If Canterbury's current leadership had taken their posts a decade earlier, it seems unlikely that the 'showcase' could have happened. Influenced by what was happening in the United Kingdom, the centre-right government of the early 1990s introduced a purchaser–provider split, recast public hospitals as independent 'crown health enterprises', and introduced financial incentives in the form of payment for activity and competition between providers for service contracts.

It is almost universally agreed in New Zealand that these reforms were a failure. The government had promised that its reforms would deliver dramatic efficiency improvements, shorter waiting lists and better control of public health spending. In practice, the regional authorities found themselves embroiled in intractable contract negotiations with the hospitals, transaction costs soared, while competition failed to develop (Hornblow 1997). In 2001, a Labour-led coalition removed the purchaser–provider split, establishing new district health boards to oversee the planning and funding of local services and to manage public hospitals.

In Canterbury, the 'showcase' in the warehouse marked the transition from a purchasing model for managing services, one with strict separation of roles, to a collaborative approach to addressing complex, system-wide challenges. It would be an exaggeration to claim that the 'showcase' delivered a detailed blueprint for redesigning services. There were commitments to delivering the right care, in the right place and at the right time. There was a pictogram with the patient's home at the centre and various services wrapped around it. What seems important is that these initiatives helped to create a sense of collective responsibility for the health system, that organisations in the system needed to act as 'one system' with 'one budget', a recognition of the need for change and a social movement in favour of transformation.

As others have argued, Canterbury's success depended on the vision, the social movement and sustained investments to support staff in delivering service change (Timmins and Ham 2013). The health board also made significant changes to the governance of the health system to support a collective approach. Rather than maintaining the traditional division of responsibilities between funders and independent providers, it asked providers to enter new a new 'alliance agreement', overlaying other contracts, in which they committed to working together to serve the best interests of the population. It invited public, not-for-profit and private providers to join an 'alliance board', chaired by a patient representative, to make decisions on use of resources and management of the system. While the health board cannot formally delegate duties to the alliance, it accepts the advice of clinicians on the alliance board on how to deploy resources to meet the population's needs, for example how to use savings or how to manage overspends.

Leaders of the health board sometimes compare their approach to alliance contracting in the construction industry. While there are some similarities, these are not the detailed agreements used to bind together the parties in some commercial joint ventures. Nor are there any complex formulae to share gains and losses between participating organisations. Instead, the aim is to create 'high trust' and 'low bureaucracy' with simple contracts.

Alongside these changes, the health board removed payment for performance and activity from its contracts with providers. Rather than engineering complex new incentive schemes, the board allocates providers an annual grant based on a bottom-up assessment of the costs of delivering services. If public or not-for-profit providers make efficiencies, the alliance decides how best to deploy these resources across the system. Private providers can make a maximum return on investment and any additional profits are given back to the system. Rather than attempting to transfer risk and reward to providers, the health board commits to ensuring the sustainability of organisations in the alliance. If a provider enters difficulty, the alliance will work with it to address the problem and reallocate resources if needed to allow it to recover. While there are occasional procurements for new services, for example laboratory diagnostics, the health board does not pitch its core group of established providers against each other in tendering competitions. Instead, there is an expectation that it will work with these partners in perpetuity.

For Carolyn Gullery, the Executive Director for Funding and Planning at the health board, these changes to payments and contracting were essential features rather than optional details of Canterbury's collaborative model. It isn't realistic for funders and providers to work in co-operative partnerships while applying the tools of arm's length contracting: tendering battles, withholding payments, transferring risk and turning away if things go wrong. She told us: 'as soon as you start talking about money and contracts, collaboration goes out of the window.'

Gullery is strongly critical of attempts to harness financial incentives in integrated systems: 'Over the years, we have put in place a whole range of complex financial incentives. They never work. In a complex system, financial incentives inevitably become perverse.' As for proposals to transfer risk to providers:

> One of the interesting things about transferring risk in these models is in fact you don't. Ultimately the risk comes back to the health board. Because if that provider fails, who is going to pick it up? We're not suddenly going to leave patients without care. So, if you step back and realise that this is about making sure you've got care for patients, you move away from these approaches and you move to a collaborative approach.

Bolton Foundation Trust

In April 2012, Monitor placed Bolton Foundation Trust in breach of its licence conditions. The Trust had struggled to maintain quality standards and financial balance following expansion and acquisition of new services in 2011. By the spring of 2012, it had failed to meet waiting time targets for three quarters and accumulated a trading deficit of £1.9 million for the year (National Audit Office 2014). Monitor required the Trust to appoint a new interim chair and turnaround director and commission an independent review of its governance (National Audit Office 2014). At Monitor's instigation, management consultants swept in and, over the following year, charged £3.5 million to support restructuring (Bell 2013).

The new leadership at the hospital faced intense pressure from Monitor to eliminate its growing deficit and improve clinical performance. Meanwhile, Bolton Clinical Commissioning Group (CCG) faced comparable pressure from NHS England to control spending and stay in financial balance. Over the next four years, the commissioner and provider attempted to improve their respective financial positions by using Payment by Results rules. The foundation trust sought additional income to cover higher demand for particular services. The CCG countered by reviewing its billing for different services and applying penalties for missed performance standards. From 2014 to 2015, the CCG and foundation trust sent each other more than 300 formal letters in contractual disputes about activity levels, performance standards and withheld payments. Meanwhile, the big questions about the shape of the local system and how to transform services went unanswered.

By early 2016, leaders at the two organisations recognised that something needed to change. Large teams in the CCG and the hospital were distracted with contractual disputes, rather than working together to improve services. Leaders on both sides agreed that their approach to contracting and the payment system were at the heart of this way of working. The commissioner relied on ineffective contractual levers to manage the foundation trust's performance. Meanwhile the foundation trust was encouraged to drive up activity under 'payment for results' rather than making efficient use of resources. The reliance on financial incentives encouraged dissimulation and denial of responsibility.

In 2016, the two organisations agreed a set of very simple principles for how they wanted to work together. They agreed that they should:

- work in the interests of the local system rather than the interests of their individual organisations

- work collaboratively to support the transformation of services for the local population

- work openly and transparently, including by sharing information on finance and performance on an open book basis

- share risk rather than attempting to transfer it to one another

- work together to protect the sustainability of the system, considering it a failure for both organisations if either accumulated a deficit.

At the same time, they agreed to replace payment for activity with a contract value based on the costs of delivering services, with simple arrangements for sharing savings or deficits. The commissioner agrees to pay the hospital a contract value of around £200 million for the year, based on an assessment of its revenues for the previous year and expected changes in activity and costs. The commissioner and hospital will share the costs of higher than expected demand for A&E services and take joint responsibility for addressing the problem if it arises. The hospital takes greater responsibility for managing demand for other services and switching to more effective modes of delivery, retaining the savings if it does this successfully. Meanwhile, the CCG puts aside an annual budget to manage contingencies. The CCG continues to monitor the hospital's performance against requirements in its contracts and CQUIN metrics. However, it uses this data as a basis for discussions on improvement rather than grounds for making or withholding incentive payments.

Since making these changes, the CCG, hospital and other providers have been working to improve performance across the system. For example, the hospital is increasing the use of telephone appointments and virtual clinics and redesigning services to reduce reliance on hospital-based treatments, with estimated savings of £200,000 in the first year. The hospital has been able to deliver recurrent savings of over £1 million from reducing costs of expensive drugs and savings of £1 million from better estates utilisation, none of which would have been possible under the previous financing regime. The commissioner and hospital have been able to complete annual contract negotiations quickly, without protracted arguments about the impact of tariff changes, appropriate service improvement targets or approaches to counting and coding data, since their financial stability no longer depends on these details. The commissioner estimates that it has achieved a saving of £250,000 per year on contract management. Staff who used to work on disputes are now working on improvement projects.

5 End note: from contracts to collaboration

There is an urgent need to reform the system for paying and contracting for services in the English NHS. The old combination of payment for activity for hospitals and capitation or block contracts in primary, community and mental health services makes it difficult for hospitals to stop wasteful activities for fear of losing revenues, obstructs collaboration on system-wide improvement projects, and makes it harder to move resources to areas where they might deliver greatest impact such as prevention, primary care and mental health. The leaders of local systems have found themselves locked in disagreements about relatively small incentive payments, rather than focusing on the big opportunities for system-wide improvement. Significant sums have been spent devising, policing and contesting elaborate incentive schemes, for example the £9.8 million spent on the UnitingCare contract (National Audit Office 2016), sums that seem likely to outweigh any benefits that these schemes could offer in a public health system.

After thirty years of financial engineering, there is a strong temptation not simply to dismantle our current, obstructive payment mechanisms but to create new, sophisticated pay for performance schemes to replace them. A host of technical experts in national bodies, consultancies and think tanks are encouraging the NHS to do so. However, there are few reasons to believe that the new schemes being contemplated will be any more successful than their predecessors. The latest schemes are modelled on accountable care contracts in insurance-based health systems with little consideration of the fundamental differences between these systems and tax-funded public systems such as the NHS. Over recent years, NHS organisations in many parts of England – Cambridgeshire, Staffordshire, Oxfordshire among others – have already dedicated substantial resources to these types of schemes. With hindsight, insiders question whether this represented a good use of time and money.

Rather than new complex schemes, commissioners should develop simple arrangements that allow resources to be allocated where they are most needed, make it easier for organisations to collaborate on improvement and promote a culture of collective responsibility for local health systems. The aim should be to spend as little time as possible discussing payment schemes and as much time as possible collaborating on actual improvement. As in Canterbury and Bolton, this probably means moving to global budgets for providers based on a bottom-up estimate of the costs they will incur to deliver the required services. Rather than attempting to transfer risk to each other, they should agree to work together to manage risks such as increasing population need, demand for services or costs of delivering services and to ensure the sustainability of individual organisations and the system. Rather than complex gain/loss sharing agreements, organisations should decide together how best to use savings from particular improvement projects or cope with overspends.

There will be voices advocating the introduction of complexity into these systems, for example targeted incentives or the combination of block contracts with activity-based payments for some services. However, there is little space for such approaches in systems organised on these lines. Commissioners cannot usefully mix and match incentive payments, payment for activity and block contracts while committing to protecting providers' sustainability. There may of course be a continued need to pay organisations outside the system for some services on a fee-for-service basis, for example where patients are sent to external providers for specialist care.

None of this is a panacea for the immense challenges of delivering improvement in complex local health and care systems. On the contrary, it is possible that the removal of pay for activity and a return to block contracts, introduced in isolation, could lead to stricter rationing rather than faster improvement. Canterbury and other examples highlight the importance of developing vision, culture, particular styles of leadership, careful monitoring of performance and investment in improvement systems in sustaining high performance, in association with changes to payments and contracting. Nevertheless, the Bolton story and similar examples suggest that removing existing toxic incentive schemes can be a useful start, replacing them not with new complex incentives, but simple arrangements that allow local leaders to move resources where needed, reduce transaction costs, defuse hostility and work in constructive partnerships.

References

Bajari P, Tadelis S (2001). 'Incentives versus transaction costs: a theory of procurement contracts'. *The RAND Journal of Economics*, 32(3), pp 387–407.

Bell J (2013). 'Cash-strapped hospital spends £3.5 million on management consultants to solve its woes'. *The Bolton News*. Available at: www.theboltonnews.co.uk/news/boltonnews/10517883. Cash_strapped_hospital_spends___3_5_million_on_management_consultants_to_solve_its_woes/ ?commentSort=score (accessed on 8 January 2019).

Berwick DM (2013). *A promise to learn – a commitment to act: improving the safety of patients in England*. London: Department of Health. Available at: www.gov.uk/government/publications/ berwick-review-into-patient-safety (accessed on 8 January 2019).

Berwick DM (1995). 'The toxicity of pay for performance'. *Quality Management in Health Care*, 4(1), pp 27–33.

Chapman J (2004). *System failure: why governments must learn to think differently*, 2nd ed. London: Demos. Available at: www.demos.co.uk/files/systemfailure2.pdf (accessed on 6 February 2019).

Charles A (2017). *Developing accountable care systems: lessons from Canterbury, New Zealand*. London: The King's Fund. Available at: www.kingsfund.org.uk/publications/developing-accountable-care-systems (accessed on 8 January 2019).

Cottam H (2018). *Radical help: how we can remake the relationships between us and revolutionise the welfare state*. London: Virago.

Department of Health (2010). *Equity and excellence: liberating the NHS*. London: Department of Health. Available at: https://assets.publishing.service.gov.uk/government/uploads/system/uploads/ attachment_data/file/213823/dh_117794.pdf (accessed on 8 January 2019).

Enthoven A (1999). *In pursuit of an improving national health service*. London: Nuffield Trust. Available at: www.nuffieldtrust.org.uk/research/in-pursuit-of-an-improving-national-health-service (accessed on 7 February 2019).

Enthoven A (1985). *Reflections on the management of the national health service*. London: Nuffield Trust. Available at: www.nuffieldtrust.org.uk/research/reflections-on-the-management-of-the-national-health-service (accessed on 7 February 2019).

Forbes LJ, Marchand C, Doran T, Peckham S (2017). 'The role of the quality and outcomes framework in the care of long-term conditions: a systematic review'. *British Journal of General Practice*, 67(664), pp e775–e784.

Ford J, Plimmer G (2018). 'Returning the UK's privatized services to the public'. *Financial Times*. Available at: www.ft.com/content/90c0f8e8-17fd-11e8-9e9c-25c814761640 (accessed on 7 February 2019).

Gullery C, Hamilton G (2015). 'Towards integrated person-centred healthcare – the Canterbury journey'. *Future Hospital Journal*, 2(2), pp 111–116.

Ham C, Alderwick H (2015). *Place-based systems of care: a way forward for the NHS*, London: The King's Fund. Available at: www.kingsfund.org.uk/publications/place-based-systems-care (accessed on 6 February 2019).

Hood C (1995). 'The new public management in the 1980s'. *Accounting, Organizations and Society*, 20(2/3), pp 93–109.

Hood C (1991). 'A public management for all seasons?'. *Public Administration*, 69(1), pp 3–19.

Hornblow A (1997). 'New Zealand's health reforms: a clash of cultures'. *British Medical Journal*, 314(7098), pp 1892–1894.

House of Commons Transport Committee (2017). *Rail franchising* [online]. House of Commons website. Available at: https://publications.parliament.uk/pa/cm201617/cmselect/cmtrans/66/6603.htm (accessed on 7 February 2019).

Illman J (2018). 'NHS England urged to axe "perverse" cancer funding policy'. *Health Service Journal*. Available at: www.hsj.co.uk/quality-and-performance/nhs-england-urged-to-axe-perverse-cancer-funding-policy/7023094.article (accessed on 8 January 2019).

Lewis R, Agathangelou G (2018). *How should payment systems evolve in the new era of integrated care?* Blog. Nuffield Trust. Available at: www.nuffieldtrust.org.uk/news-item/how-should-payment-systems-evolve-in-the-new-era-of-integrated-care (accessed on 8 January 2019).

Marmot M (2004). 'Status syndrome'. *Significance*, 1(4), pp 150–54.

Millar F (2018). *The best for my child: did the schools market deliver?* Woodbridge: John Catt Education Limited.

Monitor (2014). *Capitation: international examples* [online]. Monitor. Available at: www.gov.uk/government/publications/capitation-international-examples (accessed on 8 January 2019).

National Audit Office (2016). *Investigation into the collapse of the UnitingCare Partnership contract in Cambridgeshire and Peterborough*. National Audit Office. Available at: www.nao.org.uk/report/investigation-into-the-collapse-of-the-unitingcare-partnership-contract-in-cambridgeshire-and-peterborough (accessed on 7 February 2019).

National Audit Office (2014). *Monitor: Regulating NHS foundation trusts*. National Audit Office. Available at: www.nao.org.uk/report/monitor-regulating-nhs-foundation-trusts-2 (accessed on 25 February 2018).

NHS England (2019). *NHS long term plan*. NHS England. Available at: www.england.nhs.uk/long-term-plan (accessed on 7 February 2019).

NHS England (2018a). *Contracting arrangements for integrated care providers (ICPs)*. NHS England website. Available at: https://www.engage.england.nhs.uk/consultation/proposed-contracting-arrangements-for-icps (accessed on 8 January 2019).

NHS England (2018b). *Incentives framework for integrated care providers (ICPs)*. NHS England [online]. Available at: www.england.nhs.uk/publication/incentives-framework-for-integrated-care-providers-icps (accessed on 8 January 2019).

NHS England (2018c). *Overview of integrated budgets for integrated care providers (ICPs)*. NHS England website. Available at: www.england.nhs.uk/publication/overview-of-integrated-budgets-for-integrated-care-providers-icps (accessed on 8 January 2019).

NHS England (2018d). *Questions and answers, draft integrated care provider (ICP) contract package*. NHS England website. Available at: https://www.engage.england.nhs.uk/consultation/proposed-contracting-arrangements-for-icps (accessed on 8 January 2019).

NHS England (2017). *Whole population models of provision: establishing integrated budgets*. NHS England website. https://www.england.nhs.uk/publication/whole-population-models-of-provision-establishing-integrated-budgets-document-7b (accessed on 7 February 2019).

PricewaterhouseCoopers (2012). *An evaluation of the reimbursement system for NHS-funded care: a report for Monitor*. London: Monitor. Available at: www.gov.uk/government/publications/the-reimbursement-system-for-nhs-funded-care-an-evaluation (accessed on 8 January 2019).

PricewaterhouseCoopers, Healthcare Financial Management Association (2018). *Making money work in the health and care system*. PricewaterhouseCooper. Available at: www.pwc.co.uk/industries/government-public-sector/healthcare/insights/making-money-work.html (accessed on 8 January 2019).

Raleigh VS (2018). 'Stalling life expectancy in the UK'. *British Medical Journal*, 362, p 4050.

Scott JC (1998). *Seeing like a state: how certain schemes to improve the human condition have failed*. New Haven: Yale University Press.

Thomas R, Dunhill L (2018). '"CQUIN should be scrapped or overhauled", say local leaders'. *Health Service Journal*. Available at: www.hsj.co.uk/finance-and-efficiency/cquin-should-be-scrapped-or-overhauled-say-local-leaders/7022815.article (accessed on 8 January 2019).

Timmins N, Ham C (2013). *The quest for integrated health and social care: a case study in Canterbury, New Zealand*. London: The King's Fund. Available at: https://www.kingsfund.org.uk/publications/quest-integrated-health-and-social-care (accessed on 6 February 2019).

Wyatt S (2018). *Risk and reward sharing for NHS integrated care systems*. The Strategy Unit. Available at: https://www.strategyunitwm.nhs.uk/publications/risk-and-reward-sharing-nhs-integrated-care-systems (accessed on 8 January 2019).

About the author

Ben is a project director at the King's Fund. His work includes research on high performing health systems, new care models, the regulation of health services and innovation.

Before joining the Fund, Ben worked as a management consultant. He has advised central government and the national bodies on a wide range of issues including economic regulation, provider finance, the provider failure regime and new organisational models. He has also worked with large numbers of NHS purchasers and providers on strategic and operational challenges.

Published by
The King's Fund
11–13 Cavendish Square
London W1G 0AN
Tel: 020 7307 2568
Fax: 020 7307 2801

Email:
publications@kingsfund.org.uk

www.kingsfund.org.uk

© The King's Fund 2019

First published 2019
by The King's Fund

Charity registration number:
1126980

All rights reserved, including the
right of reproduction in whole or
in part in any form

ISBN: 978 1 909029 91 0

A catalogue record for this
publication is available from
the British Library

Edited by Megan Price

Typeset by
Grasshopper Design Company,
www.grasshopperdesign.net

Printed in the UK by
The King's Fund

The King's Fund is an independent charity working to improve health and care in England. We help to shape policy and practice through research and analysis; develop individuals, teams and organisations; promote understanding of the health and social care system; and bring people together to learn, share knowledge and debate. Our vision is that the best possible health and care is available to all.

www.kingsfund.org.uk 🐦 **@thekingsfund**